About The Authors

GW00738527

Dr Michael J. Bulstrode is an acknowledged expert on matters sexual. There are not many things he does not know about sex, though how to satisfy his wife is one of them. Last year he went to Helsinki to set up an international commission on the prevention of sexually transmitted diseases and he has been visiting special clinics ever since.

His many books and even more appearances on TV programmes are all part of Dr Bulstrode's desire to take science to the people and money to his bank account. Dr Bulstrode has attended universities in England, America and the Cayman Islands, studied medicine with the St John's Ambulance Brigade and holds a doctorate in home economics.

Molly Black early 1960s anti-establishment iconoclast and jour-nalist. Her books, *The Female Marxist*, *No Cheers for Motherhood* and *Kill All Men*, sent shock waves through contemporary Britain and throughout the Western World.

Twenty years on she is a well-known and sympathetic agony aunt working for a number of newspapers, magazines and radio stations. But she frequently says that she has lost none of her revolutionary zeal. She lives with her husband, a London solicitor, and their three children in a converted oast house in Surrey.

SAFE SEX JUKE BOX JURY

HITS

1 **Let's Not Go To San Francisco** — *The Flower Pot Men*

2 **Love Me Don't** — *The Beatles*

3 **I Want Your Safe Sex** — *George Michael*

4 **Rubber Soul** — *The Beatles*

5 **Dominic** — *The Singing Nun*

MISSES

1 **Je T'Aime (Moi Non Plus)** — *Serge Gainsberg and Jane Birkin*

2 **My Ding A Ling (12″ version)** — *Chuck Berry*

3 **Jump Up and Down And Wave Your Knickers In The Air** — *Jonathan King*

4 **I Love Jumping Up And Down And Waving My Ding A Ling In The Air** — *Chuck King*

5 **My Little Stick Of Blackpool Euphemism** — *George Formby*

THE SAFE SEX SURVIVAL MANUAL

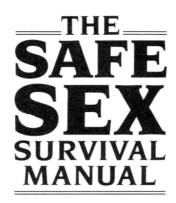

Dr Michael J. Bulstrode
and
Molly Blackburn

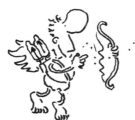

CENTURY

LONDON MELBOURNE AUCKLAND JOHANNESBURG

First published in 1987 by Century Hutchinson
Ltd, Brookmount House, 62–65 Chandos Place,
Covent Garden, London WC2N 4NW

Century Hutchinson Australia Pty Ltd, PO Box
496, 16–22 Church Street, Hawthorn, Victoria
3122, Australia

Century Hutchinson New Zealand Ltd, PO Box
40–086, Glenfield, Auckland 10, New Zealand

Century Hutchinson South Africa Pty Ltd, PO
Box 337, Bergvlei, 2012 South Africa

ISBN 0 7126 1818 X

Designed by Millions Design
Illustrated by Ian Dicks

Set in 11/12pt Rotation by Falcon Graphic Art

Printed and bound by Richard Clay Ltd, Bungay,
Suffolk

CONTENTS

Authors' Foreword

This book is intended as a handy guide to lead you through the difficult sexual era which lies ahead of us. Keep it with you at all times and in particular refer to it whenever the question of sex rears its ugly head. Not too often though, as some of the more explicit passages may cause its ugly head to be reared.

Remember, all you were taught about sex as a child – that it is a natural, healthy activity for all consenting adults to indulge in on every possible occasion – was wrong. It turns out that the priests who said it was evil and would lead to hell-fire and damnation were right after all, and are no doubt licking their lips with self-satisfaction. Though do watch out for licking your lips when you have just kissed somebody – this could well be dangerous.

Sex, of course, will never go away. It is only people you have just had sex with who go away, and often do not come back.

But when it comes to the swinging sixties and the permissive society the party is over (which was usually when the sex began).

The Safe Sex Survival Manual is for the 1980s what *The Joy of Sex* was for the 1960s and *More Pictures of Couples Having It Off* was for the 1970s. At least that is what the publishers are hoping. And who are we to disagree?

MICHAEL J. BULSTRODE

MOLLY BLACKBURN

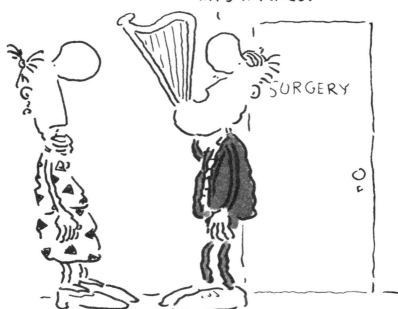

Introduction: SAFE SEX

Just as there is no such thing as a free lunch, there is no such thing as safe sex. Sex can lead to disease, pregnancy or even a long-term relationship, all of which are dangerous in their own way. At the very least it can lead to you paying for lunch.

However there are ways of making sex safer. These include:

(1) Only doing it with ONE person at a time. (Preferably yourself – see *Masturbation*.)

(2) Only doing it when fully protected by a condom, an insurance policy, the Mafia, two coats of varnish and a pair of goggles.

(3) Never doing it at all.

Bear in mind that sex is by no means the first aspect of everyday life which has been given the 'safety' treatment. Safety matches and safety razors have been with us for some time, though in neither case is the term entirely accurate. A truly safe match would not catch fire at all (and so would not be worth a light), and people frequently cut themselves on 'safety' razors. Or nearly do so, hence the expression for a near disaster, 'a close shave'.

Indeed the very use of the word 'safe' is probably tempting fate. A safe, as in 'a strong locked cupboard or cabinet for storing valuables', is only actually safe until a burglar comes along with a couple of sticks of dynamite.

The plain fact is that when God was putting the world together, He did not give a high priority to safety. Risk was the thing. So, when reading the book, do bear in mind that however much we may wish otherwise the term 'safe sex' is a relative one. And having sex with your relatives is probably one of the least safe forms of all.

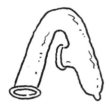

ADULTERY   Adultery is the only dangerous form of sex specifically mentioned in the Ten Commandments. (It comes just after 'Thou shalt not commit'.) The risks of having sexual intercourse with one person when you are married to someone else are obvious but fortunately there is a simple way to avoid them . . . Don't get married.

ALIMONY   One of the long-term dangers of even the safest sex, alimony is the usual American term for what most English courts refer to as 'maintenance' and what most English divorced men call a bloody nuisance.

ARSE-LICKING   Not really a sexual practice, but one of the safest ways of getting on in life in most businesses, the civil service, politics etc.

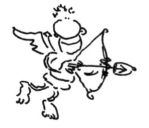

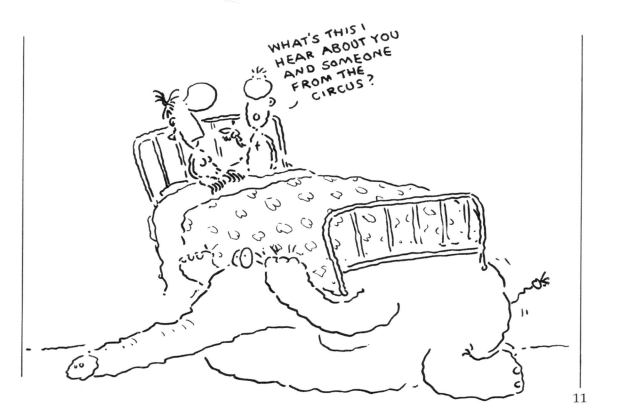

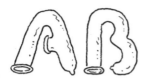

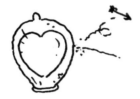

AU PAIR GIRLS Au pair girls are not usually associated with safe sex except by husbands who think their wives are *definitely* away for the weekend. (And even then they quite often turn out to be wrong.)

BONDAGE Bondage typically consists in allowing your sexual partner to chain you to the corners of a four-poster bed. This is frankly very risky indeed, depending on whose bed it is, whether they happen to be there at the time, how large the bed is and how small you are. And also whether you think your partner is to be trusted. Or trussed.

There is a certain attraction in making yourself somebody's slave (though it is not an attraction that real slaves have ever understood). But when it comes to whips, chains

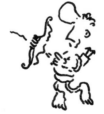

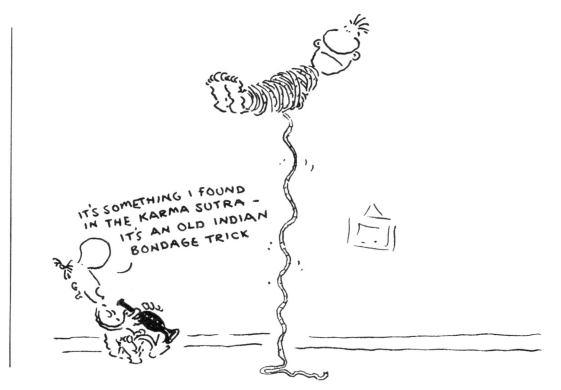

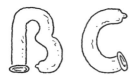

and leather – these are things to be viewed with circumspection, or better still in the pages of a porn mag.

BUNK BEDS Bunk beds provide the safest way for two people to spend all night on top of each other.

CELIBACY The safest form of sex of all, though to be honest it is more safe than sexy. Indeed if the reader has decided to opt for celibacy he need read no further, unless he wants to at least read about some of the things he is missing out on which come later in the alphabet.

Celibacy is popular with monks, nuns and priests. Or possibly unpopular with them, but at any rate they keep it up, or rather do not keep it up. It is sometimes a way of life that the rest of the world finds difficult to understand. The only thing we can confidently say

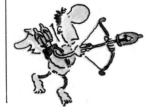

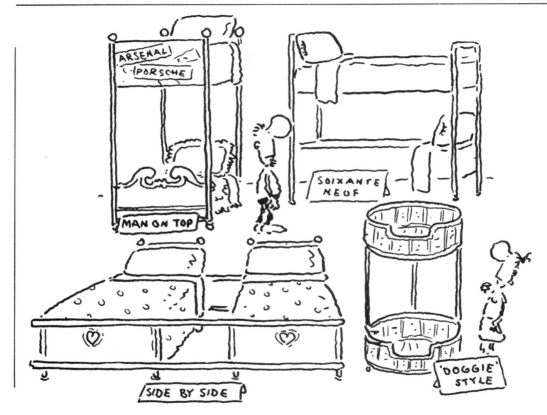

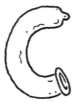

is that a desire for celibacy is not hereditary.

CHASTITY BELTS When Crusaders went to fight in the Crusades, kill the Infidel, stand around on the front of the *Daily Express* and so on, they fastened their wives into chastity belts to stop them being unfaithful while they were away. The selfish bastards did not take the trouble to hamper their own chances in the same way but most of them got killed in the fighting . . .

Thus proving that God is an Englishwoman.

Notwithstanding the horrors of the era, the time of the Crusades is looked upon as a golden age, mainly by locksmiths in fact.

COD-PIECE (1) Elaborate form of condom worn in Elizabethan times on the outside of trousers, mainly by

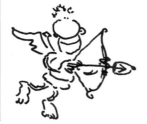

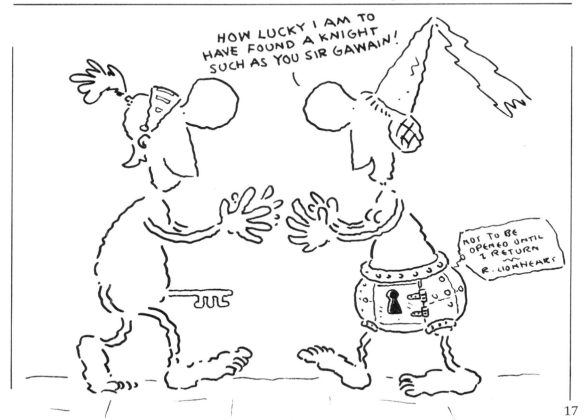

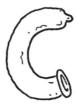

Shakespearian actors and show-offs.
(2) Slice of deep-fried foodstuff available from fish-shops.
(3) An article in *Punch*.

COLD SHOWERS Traditionally, boys at public school with surplus sexual energies are told to take a cold shower. There they are set upon by the older boys. Thus, in later life, cold showers become associated with unwelcome erections or defective hot-water systems.

CONDOMS Once the most unfashionable contraceptive since sliced bread (not that sliced bread was ever much good in that respect), the condom has bounced back as *the* contraceptive for the eighties. Its staggering return to public acceptance and esteem gives some new hope to the fight against sexually transmitted disease and even more

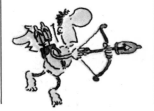

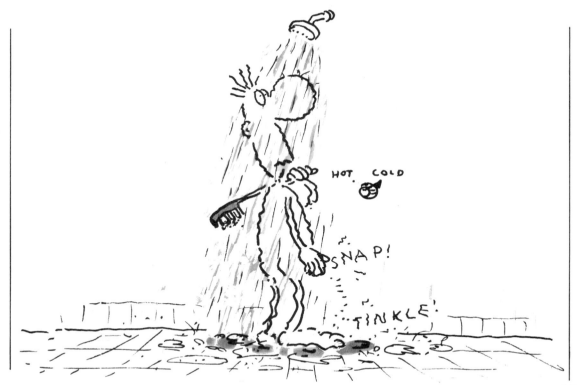

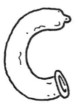

hope to other phenomena which have, unaccountably, gone out of style such as the Bay City Rollers, Simon Dee, Bear-Baiting etc.

Interestingly enough, there are many words for condom in the English language, just as there are, according to the pub bore, more than 17 Eskimo words for snow. (Useful tip for dealing with the pub bore: ask him to name *any* of them.) Condoms may be called rubbers, johnnies, French letters, Durex's, sheaths, prophylactics, etc. etc., though they are usually referred to as 'a packet of three'.

Why condoms are always sold in threes is not clear. One condom is put on the penis; where do you put the other two? What is clear is that condoms are only ever *sold* in three places:

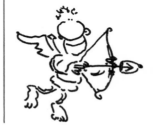

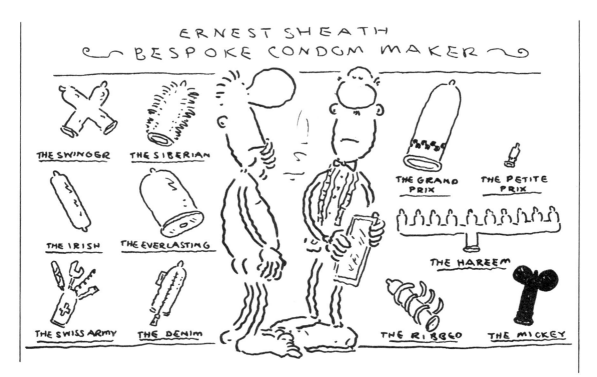

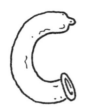

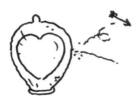

1. Old-fashioned barbers. 'Anything for the weekend, Sir?' (or is it 'weak end'?) is the traditional cry of the barber who has just made you look so unattractive that the chances of your needing a contraceptive have sunk to zero. Why barbers think that sex is something that takes place only from Friday evening to Sunday night, like London Weekend Television, is a complete mystery. (Maybe they only sleep with their wives then because they cannot stand LWT's programmes.) But if you are going to buy a weekend's worth of condoms from your hairdresser you might as well ask him for a gross. A waste of money of course but you will be treated with new respect the next time you call in to have your hair cut.

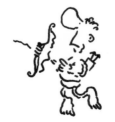

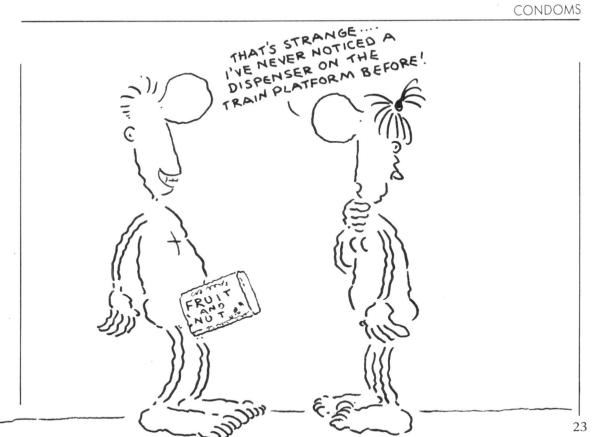

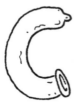

2. Chemists. Chemist shops like stocking condoms because apparently nobody ever buys *just* condoms. They always buy something else and then say, 'Oh, and a packet of Durex' (or whatever). This is very good for trade as the other thing which is bought is something that is not needed at all. Nor, it often turns out, is the condom.

3. Machines in pub lavatories. This is the best way to buy condoms as it can be done in the privacy of a smelly room with just your mates looking on and making fun of you. The only drawback is that you have to read all the endless jokes which are always written on contraceptive machines such as: *This chewing gum tastes awful, So was the Titanic, Buy me and stop one* etc.

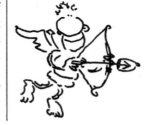

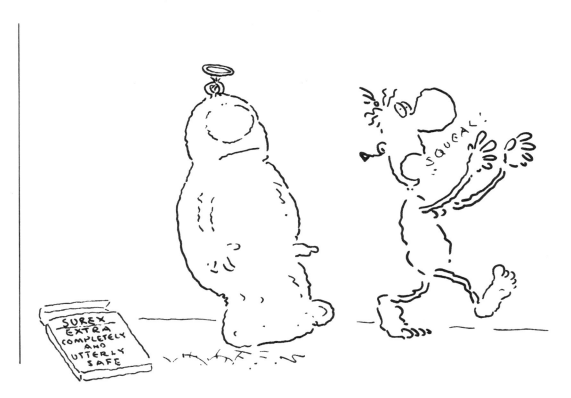

Pornographic magazines have over the years featured interviews with people whose sexual exploits have excited their readers to try to keep up . . . As our contribution to safer sex, *The Safe Sex Survival Manual* features INQUEST, the non-sex interview.

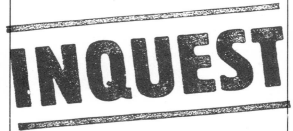

**The Laboratory of
Human Lack of Response**

INQUEST   Tell us what happened in your own words.

SALLY   Whum sploon tribby nockoes.

INQUEST   What?

SALLY   Those are just a few of my own words. I just made them up.

INQUEST   Tell us about your night of passion with Daniel (*name changed*).

SALLY   Who?

INQUEST   Daniel.

SALLY   Who's Daniel?

INQUEST   You know . . . we changed his name.

SALLY   You mean Peter?

INQUEST   Yes.

SALLY   Oh right . . . Peter.

INQUEST   Well go on then.

SALLY   OK, but as long as we call him Daniel . . . I'd be so embarrassed . . . And we mustn't call me Sally either.

INQUEST   All right, Sally. We'll call him Daniel. Go ahead.

SALLY   Well I met Peter at a party and I don't know I must have got a bit drunk or something. Or possibly I just had too much to drink. Or maybe the alcohol went to my head. Anyway I ended up doing with Peter the dirtiest thing I've ever done with a man.

INQUEST   And what was that?

SALLY   I was sick all down his trousers.

INQUEST   And so he had to take them off did he?

SALLY   I should imagine so . . . at any rate he wasn't wearing them a month later when I met him at another party. He was wearing a different pair of trousers.

INQUEST   Yes, yes . . .

SALLY   Shall I go on and tell you about this party.

INQUEST   Yes, of course.

SALLY   Only I thought you yawned . . .

INQUEST   No, no, get on with it.

SALLY   Well I had a couple of drinks at this party as well and I got chatting to Peter and he said he had to get home to his parents' house in

Chobham and I said I had a car and could I give him a lift and he said yes and, well, things just developed from there.

INQUEST   Did you go all the way?

SALLY   No, unfortunately I ran out of petrol on the Kingston by-pass, that was the problem.

INQUEST   Didn't you have a spare can?

SALLY   Yes, I got the can out of the boot and went round to the side of the car to fill it up. But it turned out I'd gone round to the wrong side of the car so I had to lean over the bonnet to get at the petrol cap and I was only wearing a short dress and as I leant over the bonnet I felt his hand go up my dress. It was, well, incredible.

INQUEST   Why was it incredible?

SALLY   Because he was 500 yards down the road in a phone box phoning the AA at the time. Anyway I heard this voice saying 'I'm going to take you right here and now on the bonnet of the car . . .'

INQUEST   This was Peter speaking.

SALLY   Yes, it must have been. I don't think the AA man could have got there as quickly as that. Anyway, he said he wanted to have sex with me there and then and, well, I said, well, you know . . .

INQUEST   Go on.

SALLY   That's right I said, 'Go on.'

INQUEST   Weren't you worried about the passing cars?

SALLY   Yes I was. They all seemed to be driving too fast and it was starting to rain and I was sure somebody was going to have an accident.

INQUEST   But you made love?

SALLY   Yes.

INQUEST   Did he use a condom?

SALLY   No, as far as I can remember he used a penis. No, I tell a lie . . . it didn't happen like this at all. I'm afraid I've been letting my imagination run away with me.

INQUEST   So you have made all of this up?

SALLY   Only the bits about running out of petrol and the sex. It was true about the parties and giving him a lift to Chobham.

INQUEST   Oh really.

SALLY   Oh, and I wasn't really sick over his trousers.

INQUEST   No?

SALLY   No, it was his shirt and tie.

INQUEST   Thank you.

SALLY   Thank you. Can I drop you off somewhere?

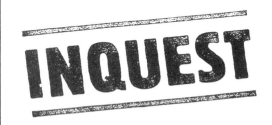

29

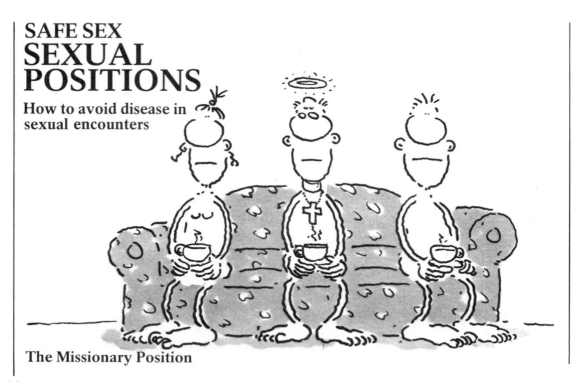

SAFE SEX
SEXUAL
POSITIONS

**How to avoid disease in
sexual encounters**

The Missionary Position

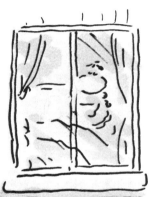

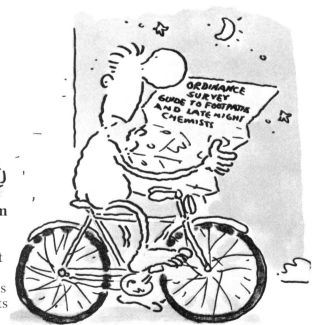

The Only if You've Got a Condom Position

Girl sits in bed while man tours neighbourhood looking for late-night chemist. Should keep you safe for a couple of hours . . . or longer if man is too embarrassed to say what he wants when he finds one

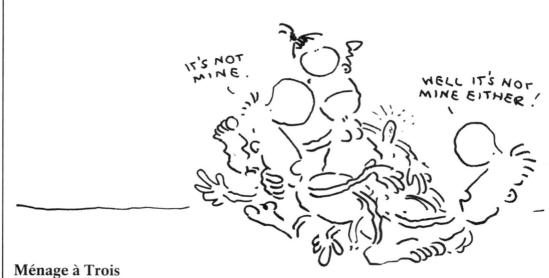

Ménage à Trois
A man with 2 women, or a woman with
2 men . . . only safe if you are not any of
them

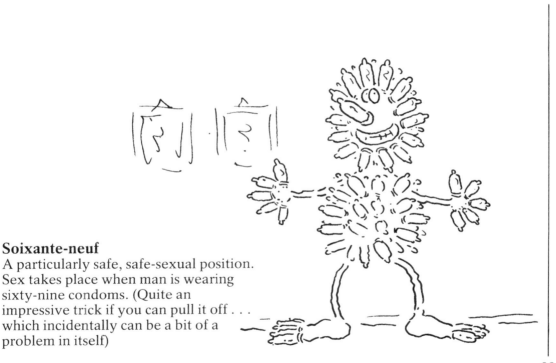

Soixante-neuf
A particularly safe, safe-sexual position.
Sex takes place when man is wearing
sixty-nine condoms. (Quite an
impressive trick if you can pull it off . . .
which incidentally can be a bit of a
problem in itself)

33

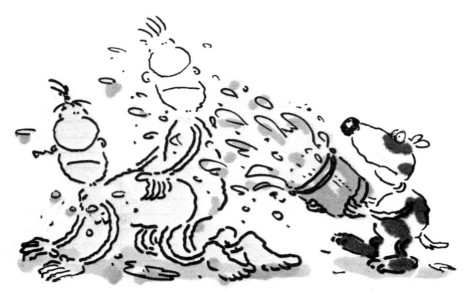

Doggy Fashion
Man enters the woman from behind;
reasonably safe for the man unless the
woman turns round

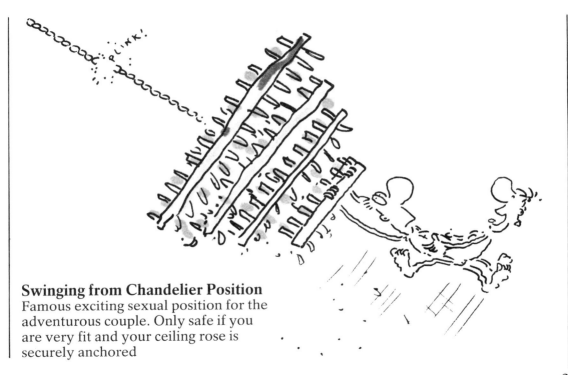

Swinging from Chandelier Position
Famous exciting sexual position for the
adventurous couple. Only safe if you
are very fit and your ceiling rose is
securely anchored

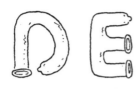

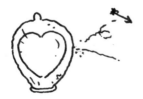

DISCOS Not to be confused with Dildos, though plenty of the one can be found in the other. It should be noted that discos are positively the worst place for getting off with possible sexual partners since with their loud music and dim light it is impossible to hear what anyone is saying or see what they look like. On the other hand for some people they are probably the best place.

EDUCATION, SEX Sex education is something all schoolchildren are exposed to a few years after learning the facts of life from their friends.

ERECTIONS These have a habit of happening at the most awkward moments such as when you are on a nudist beach or having tea with an elderly aunt (or both). They also have a habit of not happening at

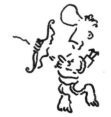

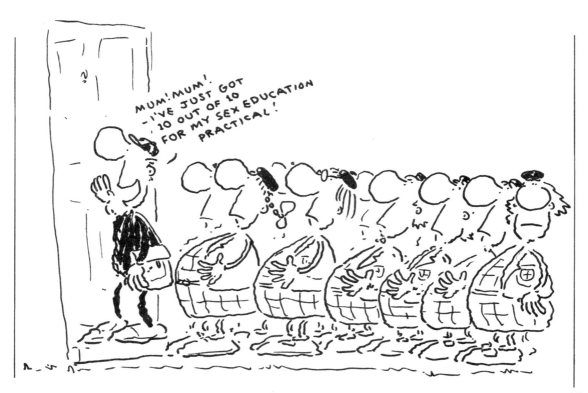

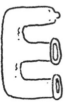

awkward moments such as just after you have got a loved one into bed after a long evening pouring gin and tonics. Strictly speaking, an erection is a rush of blood to the penis, though it usually has all the characteristics of a rush of blood to the head.

EUNUCHS Tyrants in some societies surround themselves with a harem of beautiful women and then have all the other men castrated to prevent them becoming a threat. And so make them eunuchs. On finding out how difficult it is to keep a whole harem satisfied, the tyrant probably regrets it. But the thing about becoming a eunuch, like losing your virginity, is that it's a one-way ticket. Although, if nothing else, once you have become a eunuch you are liable to

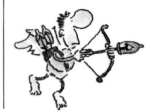

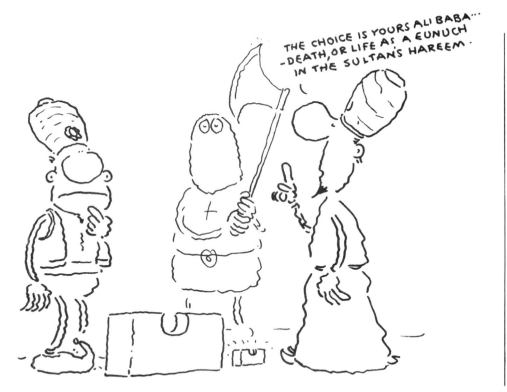

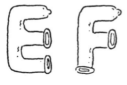

remain a virgin and avoid all the nasty diseases which might otherwise make your knob drop off. But it is nonetheless not to be recommended. It would be a bit like cutting off your nose to spite your face. Only more painful.

FLIRTING The – relatively – harmless pastime by which men and women tease each other with suggestions that they find each other sexually attractive and that actual sex might take place at any moment. To many people flirting is more fun that sex itself, rather in the way ' 'tis better to travel than to arrive', as the old British Rail slogan goes.

In fact if people confined themselves to flirting with each other and cut out the actual sex the world would be a safer place. But eventually a rather more sparsely populated

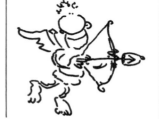

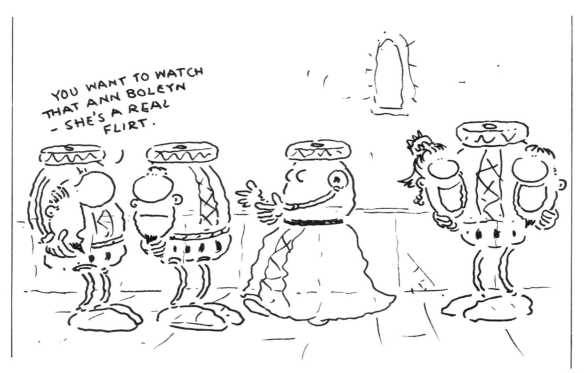

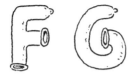

place. The sad fact is that however unsafe it becomes the world needs sex. The future of mankind needs sex. The average 15-year-old schoolboy thinks he needs sex. About 12 times a day, usually, but that's his hard luck.

FOREPLAY There was a time when foreplay was regarded as a prelude to the real thing. Nowadays it is probably safer to have a great deal of foreplay and then go straight to the post-coital cigarette, except if you do that too often you will die of lung cancer. If you do not die of frustration first, of course.

GROUP SEX One of the least safe forms of sex, particularly if the group happens to be the Beastie Boys.

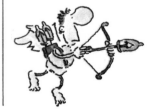

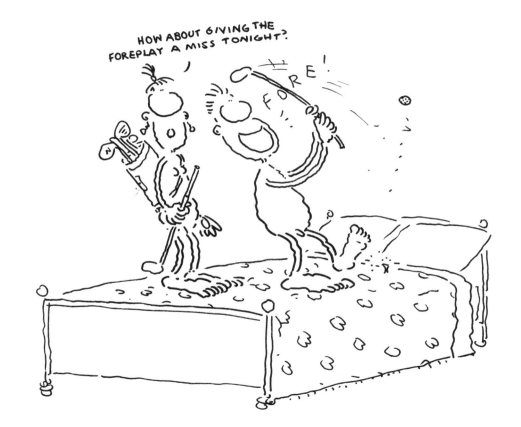

SAFE SEX FILM REVIEW

The Sound of Music II
THE SEQUEL

Julie Andrews changes her mind again and goes back to being a nun. Recommended family viewing, i.e. let your family go out and watch it while you do something more interesting (**U**).

Danish Pastry
ON THE JOB

Scandinavia's answer to Richard Hearne in workplace comedy (**14**).

Confessions Of A Maiden Aunt

Touching story of an elderly spinster in pre-war Cheltenham who confesses to returning library books late without paying the fines (**Non-U**).

LAST TANGO in TUNBRIDGE WELLS

Couple meet at the Mecca ballroom and discuss their mutual interest in dancing. Contains controversial scene with half a pound of butter, set in a Tunbridge Wells tearoom where they are taking scones and tea (**Naff**).

SORE THROAT

Linda Lovelace plays American porn movie star who catches a nasty cold and so has to stay at home sucking a Fisherman's Friend and reading the collected works of Proust **(PG)**.

9½ WEEKENDS

A man and a woman meet and he subjects her to all manner of personal indignities including 19 Arsenal League games and several day trips to his cottage in Suffolk. First acting role for Charlie Nicholas as the 'Goal-scorer' **(9½)**.

Black Emmanuelle
WASHES HER HAIR

The only night in the year in which any of the Emmanuelles does not get laid. Instead Black Emmanuelle stays in and cleans her hair with an infusion of tea **(PG Tips)**.

She's Gotta Catch It!

Black comedy about girl's sexual awakening and re-awakening, and re-awakening . . . Featuring an unbelievable number of sexually transmitted diseases **(18)**.

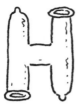

HOLIDAY ROMANCES There are many perils of foreign travel: sun burn, gippy tummy, and running into fellow Britons being just three of them.

But undoubtedly the most dangerous is the holiday romance. The combined effects of cheap flights, cheap booze and cheap thrills can be horrendous. An English girl on her first Mediterranean holiday can find herself heartbroken, pregnant and infected with an unmentionable disease as a result of one carefree fling with a handsome local.

If she manages to avoid all these disasters, there might be even worse to come: a ghastly Italian waiter turning up on her doorstep in October saying he was the one she said she loved in July and suggesting that he moves in with her for the winter.

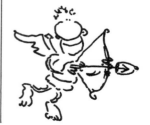

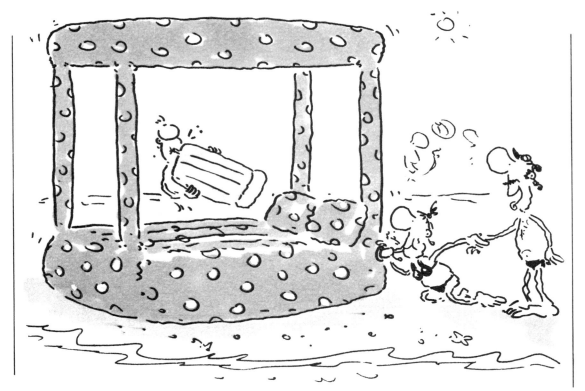

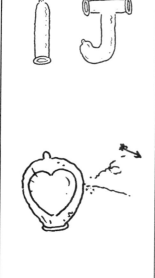

IMPOTENCE This is something that is very likely to come to most middle-aged men (unlike attractive young girls). Impotence can be very distressing but it is worth re-membering that it is not the end of the world. It is just the end of your sex-life. Surveys reveal that 5% of men suffer from impotence. Or more than 5%, depending on the size of their penis.

INTERRUPTUS, COITUS The in-genious method used by the Romans to interrupt their coiting.

JACUZZIS Warm, bubbly and satisfying – that is what the ideal girl is like when you have softened her up by sharing a jacuzzi with her. Indeed jacuzzis, like saunas, hot tubs and holidays in nudist camps are all basically ex-cuses for looking at naked people

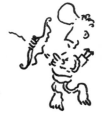

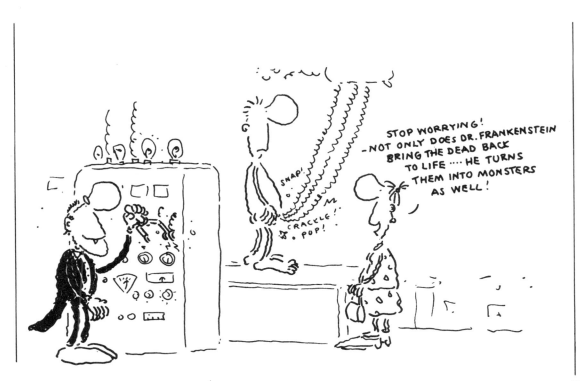

JKLM

with no blame attached, and of course no clothes attached. The defence which is advanced for the bizarre behaviour of jumping into a jacuzzi with perfect strangers without their clothes on is that it is perfectly natural and everybody does it. Which is what people used to say about bull-baiting and burning witches.

But is it dangerous?

The doctors' answer is that they think not at the moment, but they are working on it.

KISSING See under *Mistletoe*.

LIBIDO Something found in Venice, usually on a dirty weekend.

MASTURBATION Masturbation was once described as 'the thinking man's television'. This was of course before Channel 4 came along and made it possible for both activities

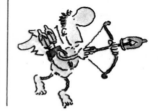

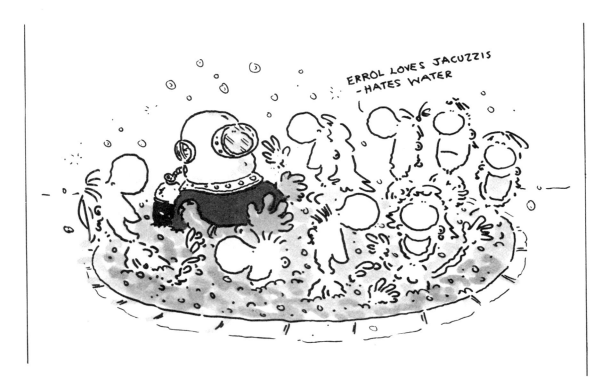

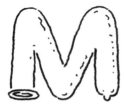

to be combined. (Thinking and television, that is.)

Masturbation is completely safe and not something to be ashamed of at all unless anybody finds out that you do it. Also makes you go blind. The great thing about masturbation is that it gives you great scope for imagination – i.e. imagining how much more satisfying real sex can be.

MISTLETOE A parasite of apple and other trees, the mistletoe plant features in human affairs at Christmas when it is hung up for people to kiss under. Nobody understands why you should kiss under the mistletoe but then nobody complains since kissing is one of the safest forms of sexual contact. From it you can usually only catch cold sores, herpes and glandular fever. Also colds, influenza, bad breath etc.

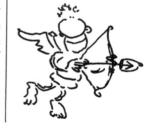

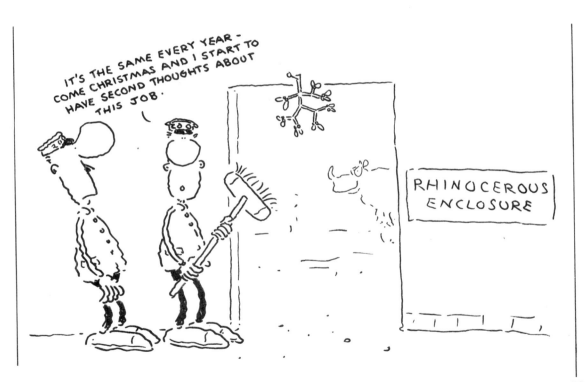

THINGS IT IS _NOT_ SAFE TO HAVE SEX WITH

Sheep When shepherds watched their flocks by night, they weren't always thinking about wolves attacking them. In fact there is a long and dishonourable tradition of lonely farming folk getting over-attached to their livestock one way or another. This is inexplicable to city dwellers who may behave like animals to each other but generally behave themselves with animals. If you _must_ have sex with sheep (although the law in fact says you _mustn't_), you should bear in mind you can catch all the usual sexually transmitted diseases plus foot-rot, sheep-tick and a hatred of mint sauce.

Hoovers Believe it or not there are some men who get their rocks off on Hoovers. (Sometimes literally, if they push things too far.) The main attraction is obviously the suction but generally the man ends up dusty and with the housework still to do. On the other hand it is absolutely heaven for the Hoover.

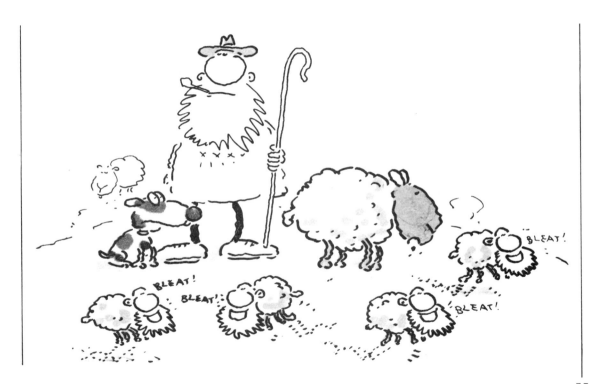

An Inflatable Rubber Woman Highly dangerous. One prick and an inflatable rubber woman can blow up in your face. Or vice versa.

Milk Bottle Even more dangerous, especially if the tits are pecking at the top at the same time

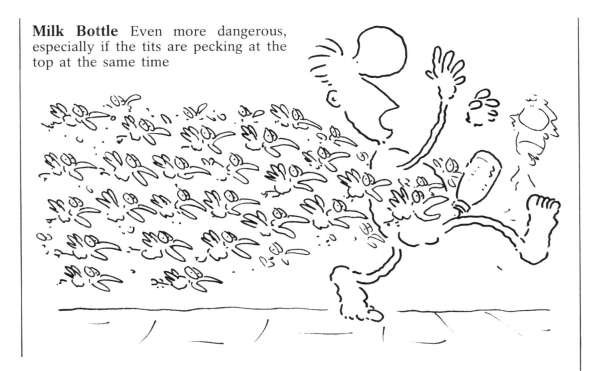

Another Human Being The most dangerous of the lot for reasons set out in this book, every newspaper you have read for about 18 months, most TV documentaries etc.

STATE OF EMERGENCY
H.M. GOVNT. DIRECTIVE

THE COMPULSORY USE
OF BARBED WIRE
UNDERWEAR
AND WARNING
BEACON
FOR ALL ADULTS
OVER THE AGE
OF 16 YEARS

THINGS IT *IS* SAFE TO HAVE SEX WITH

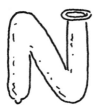

NSU Non-specific urethritis. If you go to the doctor and tell him you have got unpleasant symptoms in the area of your waterworks but you do not know what is causing them, the doctor could well tell you that you are suffering from non-specific urethritis which is a medical term meaning unpleasant symptoms in the area of the waterworks of unknown cause. Such are the wonders of medical science. NSU is yet another disease or group of diseases you get by having sexual intercourse. It's also the name of a make of car which perhaps ought to be changed for marketing in the English-speaking world. Of course the same could be said about that French fizzy drink with a name that sounds like 'Shit' and 'Ayds', the extremely unfortunately named slimming product.

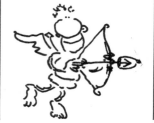

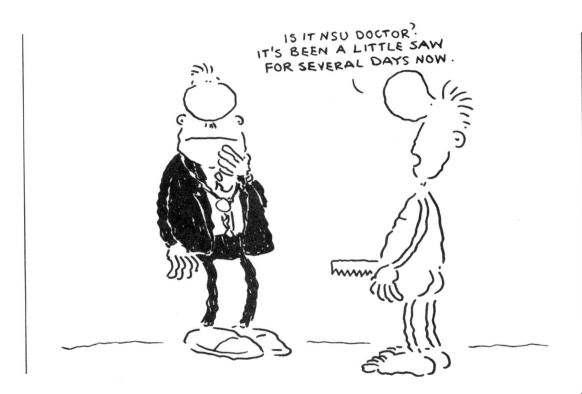

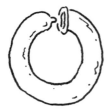

ONE-NIGHT STANDS   These can be great fun, and when you have had a really good one-night stand your first instinct is to repeat the experience. Unfortunately this is not possible, since it then becomes a two-night stand.

One-night stands are for obvious reasons very dangerous unless you take careful precautions. The most important of which being the precaution of writing down your partner's name somewhere so you get it right in the morning.

ORAL SEX   Surveys of sexual behaviour in the Western world reveal that 80% of people asked claim to indulge in mouth-to-genital contact with one or more sexual partners on a regular basis. This demonstrates the immense popularity of the main form of oral sex, i.e. talking about it.

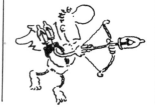

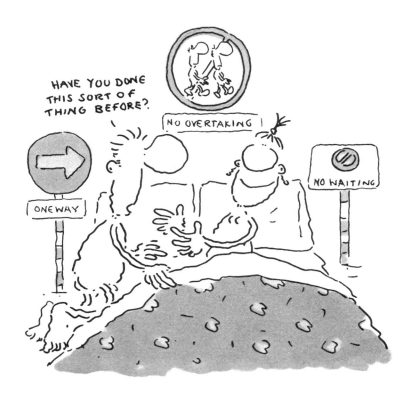

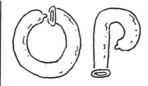

Oral sex is about as dangerous as any other form of sex except it will not make you pregnant unless you do it under a gooseberry bush with a stork.

PAGE 3 GIRLS   Page 3 Girls are the nearly naked girls whose pictures appear in a certain type of tabloid newspaper, usually on a particular page (page 3). Looking at them is a fairly safe if rather unsatisfying way of getting sexual enjoyment (but see *Masturbation*). The main danger being the possibility that you might read the newspaper which surrounds them.

PREMATURE   EJACULATION Premature ejaculation was once regarded as something to be mildly ashamed of but it is now seen as a way of keeping sex safe, depending how prematurely you manage to do

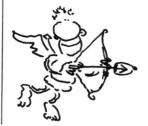

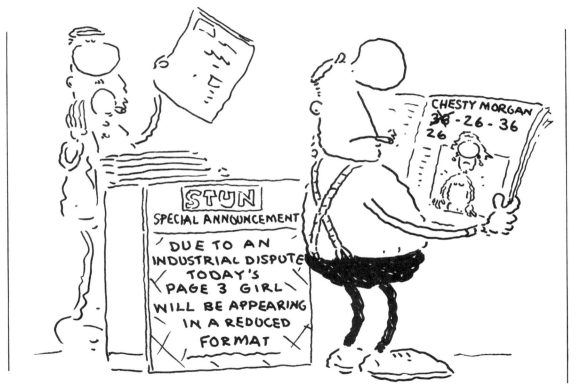

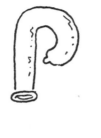

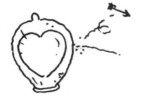

it. Ideally, this should be as early as possible, even before you arrive to pick up your date.

PROSTITUTION Prostitution is said to be the world's oldest profession and many a street-walker does look as if she has been around for quite some time. Because of their life-style prostitutes have always faced great dangers: being grabbed by the fuzz and being squeezed by their pimps are just two of them. Why then do prostitutes continue to ply their trade?

In a recent survey . . .
25% of prostitutes said they were forced into such work by poverty, desperation and the need to make ends meet.
20% said they liked working with people and liked to make ends meet.

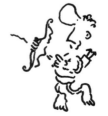

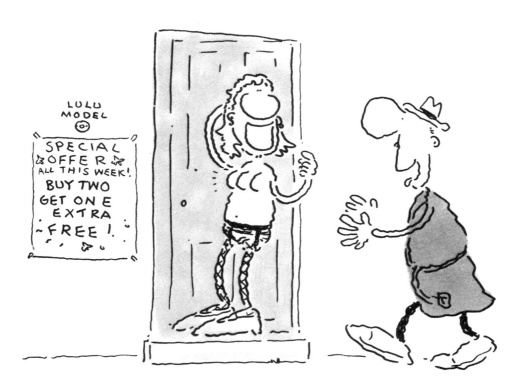

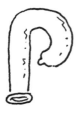

15% said they did not want to work in a factory or office. They liked working in the open air, on street corners, behind gas works, on the back seat of Ford Cortinas and so forth.

20% said they did it to avoid watching frightening TV documentaries about the spread of deadly sexually transmitted diseases.

10% said they would do anything for money. And that's £15 please for helping fill in your form, dearie. £30 without the rubber.

10% did not say anything at all because they were giving the researcher a blow job.

PUBIC LICE One of the real comedians of the natural world, the pubic louse makes his home in pubic hair, irritating the hair's owner by inflicting little bites and scuttling

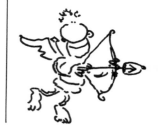

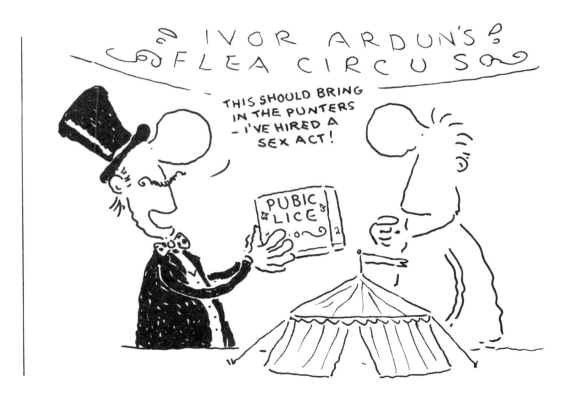

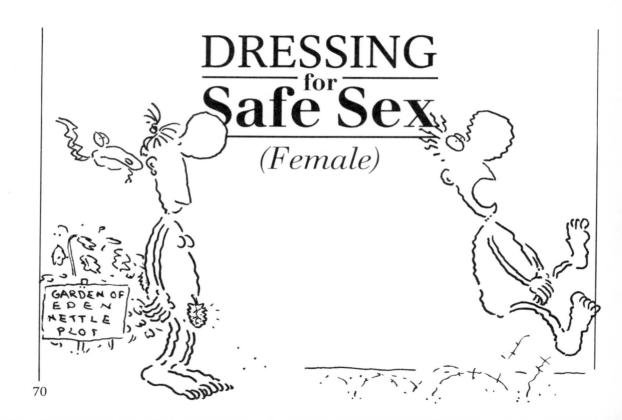

Lace-up corset
The more untying the better, since it is always possible that his ardour will cool down when faced with the laborious process of taking all this off; alternatively, it may put him in mind of lacing up football boots and he will remember Match of the Day is on.

Sheer stockings
Scarcely a turn-off but useful for tying a knot around his penis if he starts to get excited.

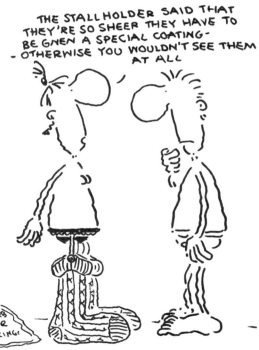

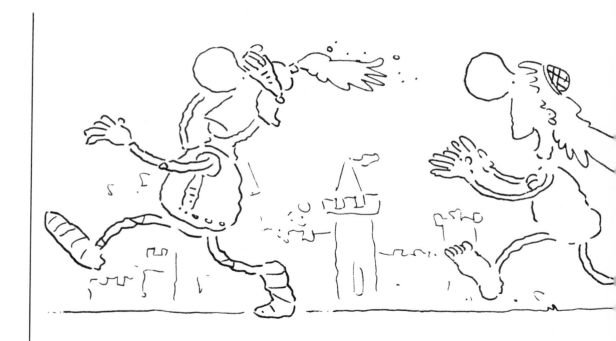

Sensible shoes
Reminds him of what his nanny used to wear and renders him temporarily impotent; also useful for kicking him in the crotch which will have the same effect.

Wedding ring
Sometimes dampens the ardour of another man; sometimes has the same effect on husband.

Chastity belt

Virginity braces

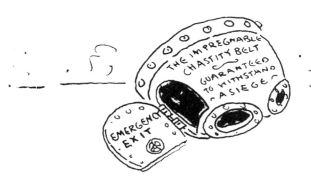

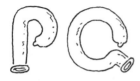

around like a thing possessed if attacked with a comb, fly swat or whatever. Pubic lice can only spread when one lot of pubic hair comes in close contact with another lot and so it does not take a great deal of working out to realise how you can catch them. Pubic lice are often referred to as crabs, though oddly enough crabs are never referred to as pubic lice.

They can be killed quite easily by a range of proprietary chemicals, by hitting them on the head or by getting little boys to catch them and put them in a bucket at the sea-side.

PUBLIC SCHOOL SEX See under *Cold showers*.

QUICKIES See *One-night stands, Knee-tremblers, Premature ejaculation*.

'Quickie' is also a type of divorce

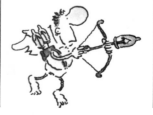

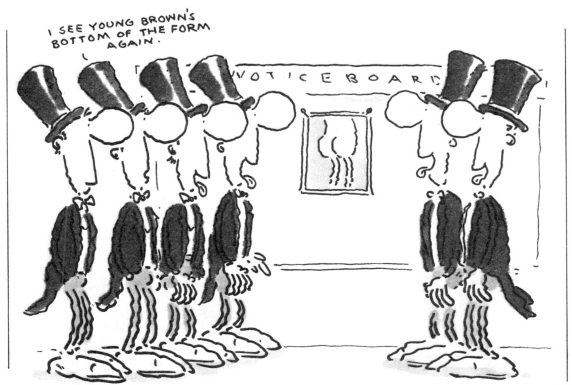

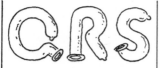

which is likely to be instituted by a wife whose husband indulges in too much of the above.

RENT BOYS Many people have never heard of Rent Boys. Anyway that is what they say when the reporter from the *News of the World* asks them about it.

Having sex with Rent Boys is not very safe. In particular:

(1) It is illegal.

(2) Rent Boys will probably blackmail you or go to the papers if you are the slightest bit rich or famous.

(3) They quite often turn nasty and cut you up with a knife and steal all your money.

Other than that it is probably perfectly all right.

SCHOOLGIRLS Many older men are unaccountably turned on by the sight of a woman dressed as a

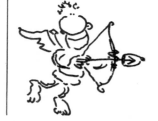

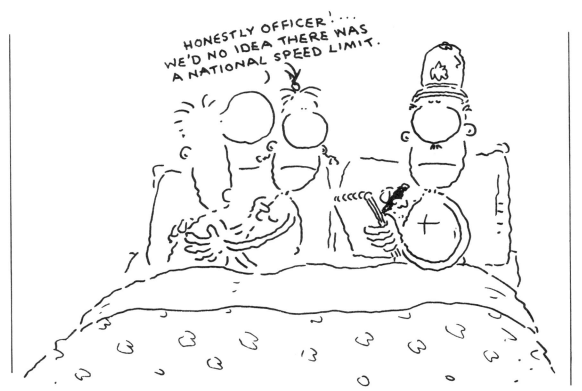

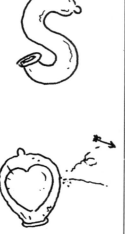

schoolgirl, or a schoolgirl dressed as a schoolgirl or, in extreme cases, a schoolboy dressed as a schoolboy. Why the appearance of a schoolgirl should be so alluring is somewhat of a mystery. It certainly puzzles the average schoolboy who will only go for a real schoolgirl if she makes herself look much older than she really is. But this perhaps demonstrates the average schoolboy's immaturity. Sex with a schoolgirl is definitely NOT safe. It probably means that she has a large crush on you and almost certainly means her father will put an even larger crush on your testicles if he ever finds out what you are up to.

Male teachers often find themselves adored by 14- or, 15-year-old schoolgirls eager to go to bed with 'Sir' . . . which is something worth

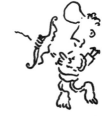

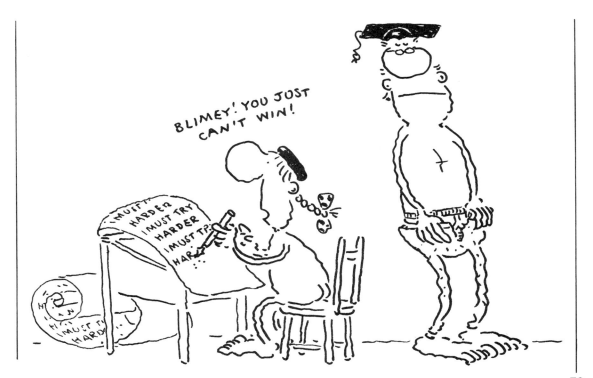

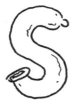

pointing out, like the long holidays and the short hours, whenever the NUT ask for a pay rise.

SEXUAL CHEMISTRY This was said to exist between David Frost, Anna Ford and Angela Rippon when TV-AM started. Whether it did or not is open to question but it certainly was not safe. They all lost their jobs within months.

SHOTGUN WEDDINGS In the pre-permissive age it was common to be forced to have a shotgun wedding if you got pregnant when unmarried. An extreme form of retribution by any standards, since shotguns make notoriously bad husbands.

SPANKING Spanking is something that happens to schoolboys when they are naughty and it is only later in life that it provides a sexual thrill. Even then it is associated with

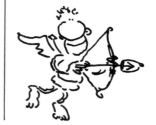

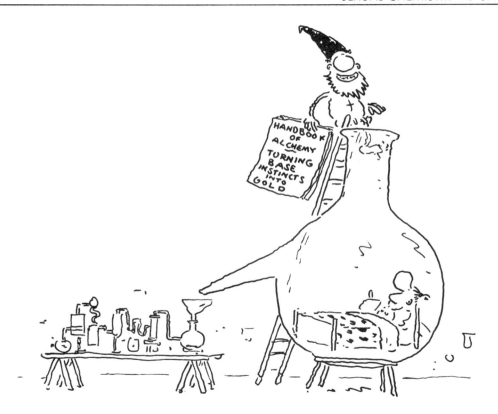

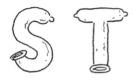

punishment, and schoolboys, and guilt. In particular if you are found guilty of spanking schoolboys you are likely to be punished. In England the punishment can be very severe, normally involving the *News of the World* camping in your front garden for months on end and your political career in ruins.

STD (1) Sexually transmitted diseases. See *VD clinics*.

(2) Subscriber trunk dialling. See *Telephone sex*.

TELEPHONE SEX This is not literally having sexual intercourse with a telephone (except in some specialist establishments in Berlin). In fact, telephone sex is the business, already booming in America, which allows frustrated businessmen to telephone a special number and hear dirty talk from a woman or

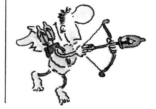

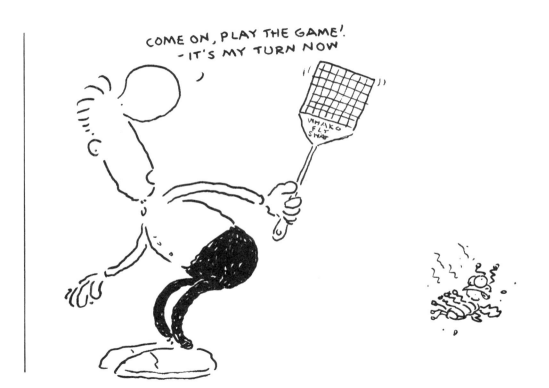

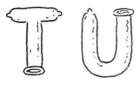

a tape recorder. Payment for the service is usually made by credit card, and the man's flexible friend can become less flexible as the call goes on. Telephone sex has the advantage of being totally safe until your wife works out why your phone bill is so high.

THRUSH An unpleasant organism which can make life very uncomfortable, especially for the worms it pecks at in the garden.

UNDERAGE SEX Parliament has decided that girls under 16 years of age are incapable of consenting to sexual intercourse, which is probably how MPs remember it from their schooldays. Despite the heavy penalties that can be imposed for having sex with young girls there is quite a lot of it that goes on. See under *Bill Wyman*.

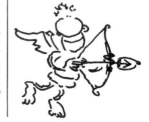

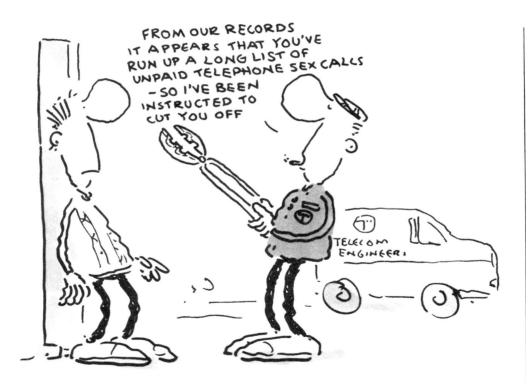

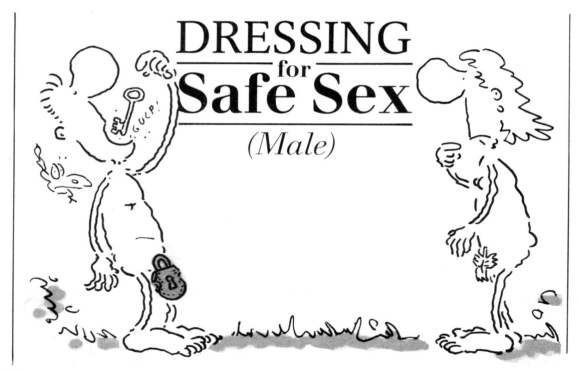

Condom on willy
(just in case)

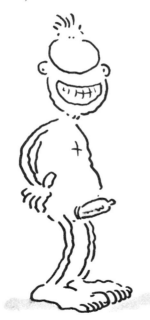

Condom in case
(also just in case)

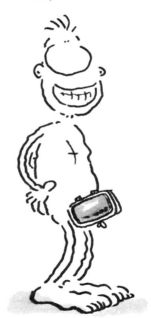

Brut aftershave
Implies either an irrational admiration for sporting celebrities like Henry Cooper or desperate desire to use up unwanted Christmas presents. Either way a turn-off.

Acrylic pullover
Sparks fly when trying to get this off in a hurry.

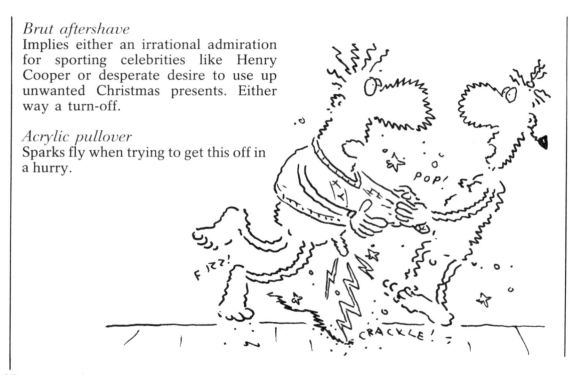

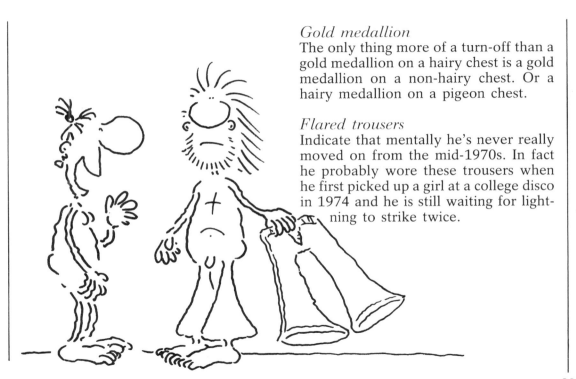

Gold medallion

The only thing more of a turn-off than a gold medallion on a hairy chest is a gold medallion on a non-hairy chest. Or a hairy medallion on a pigeon chest.

Flared trousers

Indicate that mentally he's never really moved on from the mid-1970s. In fact he probably wore these trousers when he first picked up a girl at a college disco in 1974 and he is still waiting for lightning to strike twice.

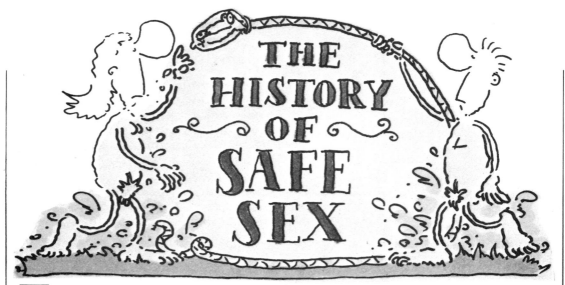

THE HISTORY OF SAFE SEX

The origins of safe sex can be traced back to the Garden of Eden where Adam and Eve wore fig leaves for protection. As a contraceptive the fig leaf did not work which was fortunate for Cain and Abel (more fortunate for Cain than Abel, as things turned out) and for the rest of us.

We think of the condom as a 20th-century item but in fact, like paper and gun-powder, it was invented five thousand years ago by the Chinese. Indeed the first condoms were actually made out of paper and gun-powder, giving rise to the expression 'the Big Bang'.

Before the discovery of rubber (in rubber trees, rubber plants and pencil erasers), condoms were made out of a variety of substances . . . leather, snakeskin and pigs' bladders being frequently employed. All were highly successful in cutting down on pregnancy as, for example, pretty well no woman wanted to have sex with a tumescent pig's bladder.

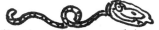

The realisation that sexual intercourse could spread disease as well as expand the population came slowly. For one thing there were so many other diseases raging that there was no particular reason to pay attention to sexually transmitted infections. After all, if it was possible to be struck down without warning by bubonic plague, why worry about a touch of gonorrhoea which was at least fun to catch?

But sexually transmitted diseases of all sorts began to arrive in Europe, brought back to the Old World by soldiers and travellers and missionaries to the New. 'Hands Across the Sea' was to come later. For a while it had been simply 'Legs Over the Natives'.

Of the diseases available, syphilis was the worst, causing its victims to go raging mad, usually with the person who gave it to them. It was known in the 17th, 18th and 19th centuries as a deadly disease which you caught by having promiscuous sex. There was no real cure. The effect on sexual behaviour was incalculable. Or, to put it another way, non-existent.

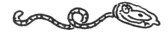

The great breakthrough in the treatment of syphilis was made by Sir Alexander Fleming. Fleming was working at St Mary's Hospital, Paddington, and noticed that a bottle of milk left on his doorstep for three weeks began to grow an interesting mould. This led to an important discovery . . . that his milkman had died. But he also discovered penicillin, too late to help his milkman, but just in time to save a few million soldiers, sailors and airmen who picked up a variety of claps and poxes in the course of the war.

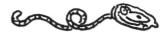

Penicillin and other antibiotics have transformed the treatment of these sexually transmitted diseases which are caused by bacteria, rendering frequent, indiscriminate sexual activity possible

. . . and leaving the way open for deadly and totally untreatable viruses. And the rest of course is history, or rather, the future.

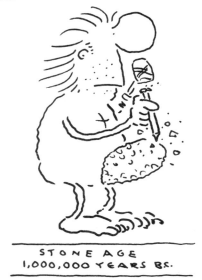

STONE AGE
1,000,000 YEARS BC.

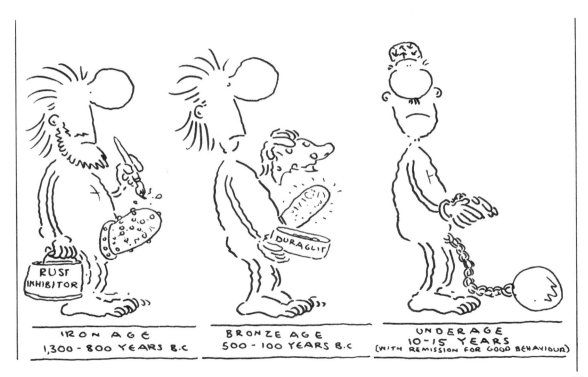

People You Shouldn't Have Sex With:
*A Girl's Guide**

Your Boss

Pretty young secretaries sometimes find themselves attracted to their boss, but anybody older and wiser would advise them not to do anything about it. Anybody older and wiser than their boss, at any rate, who will probably be strongly in favour of the idea.

Sex in the office disrupts the working routine and attracts unpleasant comments from colleagues, especially if the office is open plan.

Also, when the shit hits the fan, and his wife finds out, or you and the shit fall out, or whatever . . . who is it that gets the sack? Who is left holding the baby? Who gets forgotten? . . . Well, just you ask Cecil Parkinson's ex-secretary, whatever her name is.

Your Tutor

Sleeping with your college tutor as a way of getting through your exams is a pretty short-sighted thing to do, though it probably will help if you are short-sighted judging by the appearance of

---

* i.e. a Guide for Girls, NOT *A Girl Guide*, though incidentally having sex with a girl guide is not to be recommended. Certainly it is not a good idea to even mention to Brown Owl afterwards.

most tutors. It may get you the quali-
fications you want; it may get you the
job you want. But what happens when
your employer realises you are not as
bright as your results suggest you are?
Oh well, you can always sleep with him
as well ... (but see dangers of *Your
Boss* above).

Your Sister's Boyfriends
Girls often sleep with their sister's boyfriends. It is a natural enough competi-
tive urge that makes a girl think that if
her sister's boyfriend is attracted to *her*,
I wonder if he is attracted to *me*. And it
is not surprising that, a bit drunk at
some party or other, this urge gets fol-
lowed through. Unfortunately this
actually proves nothing. Most boys will
sleep with more or less anyone given
the opportunity, particularly when a bit
drunk at a party.

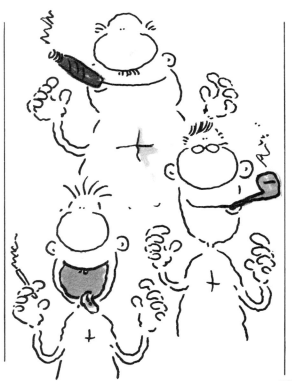

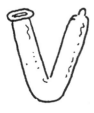

VD CLINICS   VD clinics are where you go to find out if you have caught a venereal or sexually transmitted disease. They can be difficult to find as they are never called 'VD clinics'. To spare any blushes they are called 'special clinics' or some such totally impenetrable pseudonym. Not great places for picking up a sexual partner.

VIRGINITY Virginity is something of an outmoded concept in the modern world as in the old joke:
Why wasn't Jesus born in Ireland? Because they couldn't find three Wise Men and a Virgin.
But in the new safety-conscious eighties, virginity is probably worth holding on to and there could well be a return to the idea of a girl saving herself. At least until she has sex for the first time.

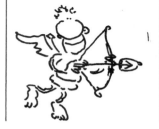

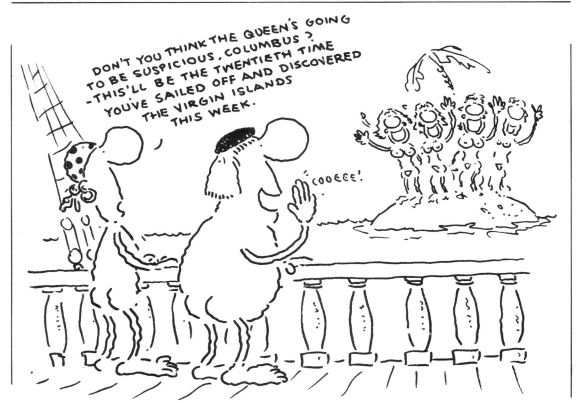

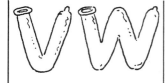

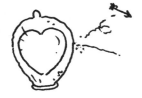

VOLVOS Not a safe form of sex but a well-known make of car which is a by-word for safety on account of its robust construction which prevents the car from crumpling in the event of a collision with a Mini, say, or a Chieftain tank. This has the effect of making Volvo drivers unusually pushy and selfish on the road. Though oddly enough, not in the least bit sexy.

VOYEURS See *Sexual antics of others*.

WIFE SWAPPING Wife-swapping is not to be recommended, especially if you are not married. Indeed, even if you are married, the concept of 'swapping' your wife temporarily for another has a definitely male chauvinist pig-like ring to it. So better call it 'husband-swapping' or 'spouse-interchanging'

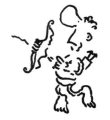

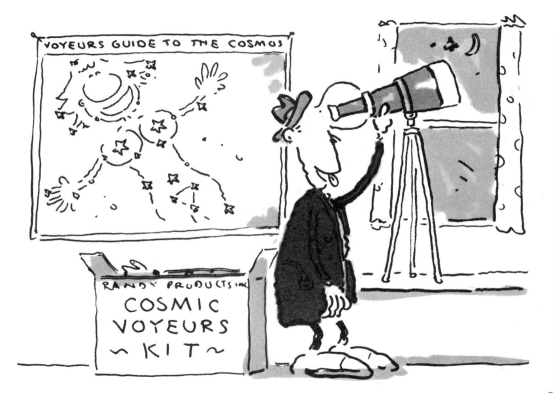

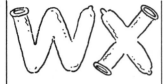

if you want to get away with it. But bear in mind that when indulging in promiscuous sex with even very close friends and neighbours, the risk of disease is ever present. If you think about it, tossing car keys on the floor and getting the women to pick them up as a way of deciding who sleeps with whom has all sorts of dangers. So do at least disinfect the car keys.

X-FILMS X-films are sometimes called 'adult movies' because they usually deal with adultery and related topics. A visit to the cinema used to be the teenager's first introduction to sex, and jolly cramped it was too. Nowadays if you see a film featuring nothing but promiscuous sex, you are likely to get a message from Bob Geldof or someone telling you how dangerous it all is. Much

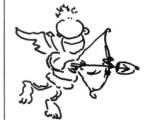

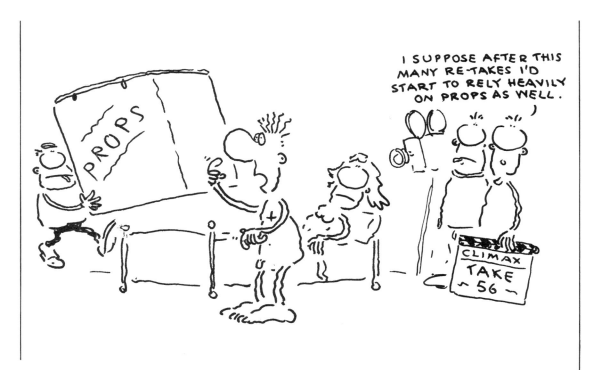

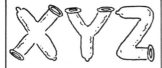

better to avoid sexy films altogether and only watch safe films . . . See *The Safe Sex Film Review* . . .

Y-CHROMOSOME The Y-chromosome is what contains a man's essential 'maleness' (or are we thinking about his Y-Fronts?).

On the Y-chromosome is programmed the genetic information for all the features special to being a man. These include testicles, a beard, a deep voice, a beer belly, receding hair, football hooliganism, wolf-whistling, arm-wrestling, smegma, Marks & Spencer ties, driving cars at 85 mph in built-up areas, wife battering, child molesting, rape, pillage and GBH. And men with 2 Y-chromosomes are even worse.

ZZZZZ . . . The sound of sleep . . . much the safest thing to do in bed, on your own or with anyone else.

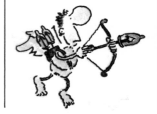

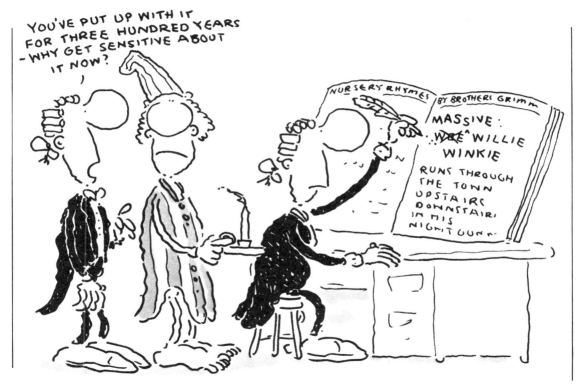

SAFE SEX THROUGH THE AGES

1)Stone Age

First human society after the Big Bang, so-called because the primitive, uncultured and selfish men of the time bore an uncanny resemblance to the modern City stockbroker.

Sex was far from safe especially for women who were invariably hit on the head with a large club as part of the courting ritual. Hence the expression 'Not tonight dear, I've got a headache.'

2) Iron Age

The discovery of iron – a valuable tool – freed primitive man from the misery of having to wear crumpled animal skins and stay-prest trousers.

Men and women died very young and consequently had sex, safe or unsafe, as often as possible as if their lives depended on it. Or as if they were on a Club 18–30 holiday.

3) Bronze Age

Nothing happened during this age but it was awarded the bronze for coming third.

4)Rubber Age

Discovery of the condom, which meant that for the first time cavemen and women could take reasonable precautions when they developed the urge to go to bed together after a couple of gin-and-tonics.

5) Ice Age

No perceivable effect on sex but useful for the gin-and-tonics.

6) Roman Empire

Era of straight roads and kinky sex, both of which were to be forgotten in England for hundreds of years until the founding of Milton Keynes, which was not built in a day, but looks as though it might have been.

7) Dark Ages

The fashion developed for having sex with the lights switched off, which was very easy as electricity had not been invented. Sex with the candle extinguished was also popular ('a blow-out job').

Increased risk of sexual disease. Increased risk of not having the first idea who you were sleeping with.

8) Renaissance (Literally, re-naissance.)

An age of re-awakening and doing it again before breakfast.

9) Tudor Age

Dominant figure was Henry VIII who was famous for having at least six sexual partners, several of them foreign, i.e. rather like spending a couple of weeks at an international conference.

This lifestyle was very risky for Henry and even more so for his wives who developed life-threatening symp – toms such as having their heads cut off.

10) Tudor Age – II

In reaction to her father's excesses Elizabeth decided to remain the Virgin Queen. She liked Essex but disliked the idea of sex. (Rather the feeling you might get looking at Graham Gooch on a rainy Tuesday at Chelmsford. Apart from liking Essex, that is.)

11) Puritan Age

Under the rule of Oliver Cromwell

England was plunged into an era of misery and restrictions when public entertainment was banned and all the theatres closed. Very similar to Shaftesbury Avenue the summer after the Americans bombed Libya. (See *No Sex Please We're British*, which is all that was on.)

12) Age of Reason

An age of enlightenment when people finally realised how boring being a Puritan was. Necklines plunged and huge bosoms were the fashion, making most men look ridiculous.

13) 19th Century

Age of prudery. Age of the Pitts. Age of people saying 'All this prudery is the pits.'

Later came Queen Victoria whose catchphrase was 'We are not amused',

soon to be adopted by millions of people forced to watch the Bob Monkhouse Show.

14) Jazz Age

The very long time it seems to take to play any piece of jazz music.

15) 20th Century

Finally the modern age. Randy men being spurned by over-modest girls were at last able to use the chat-up line 'But for Christ's sake we're living in the 20th century. And besides, your parents aren't due back till Sunday.' Sex became more widespread; so did sexual diseases.

16) Swinging Sixties

Age of wife-swapping. First recorded instance of Car Boot Sale. Also Old Boot Sale. People started to 'let it all hang out', though in other respects attitudes to laundry didn't change.

17) 1980s
The age when we all started to regret the swinging sixties. The New Puritanism began to set in. Chastity became all the rage. Nobody had any sex whatsoever.

On second thoughts, the age when we all started to regret that the swinging sixties were over.

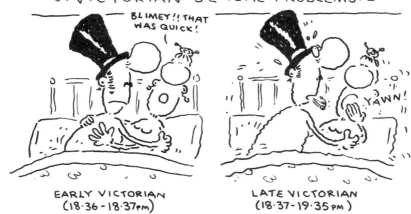

ROTHERBIE'S GUIDE TO THE DATING OF
~ VICTORIAN SEXUAL PROBLEMS ~

EARLY VICTORIAN
(18·36 - 18·37 pm)

LATE VICTORIAN
(18·37 - 19·35 pm)

ON THE LINE

Transcript of the popular radio programme in which Molly Blackburn deals with listeners' sexual and emotional problems bluntly, directly and frankly. Frankly rather unsympathetically.

CALLER   Hello Molly.

MOLLY   Hello Caller.

CALLER   It's Stephen . . .

MOLLY   Oh well, hello Stephen.

CALLER   No, it's Stephen I'm ringing about. He's my boyfriend.

MOLLY   Tell me all about it, lovie. Don't be afraid to be blunt and direct.

CALLER   Well, Molly, I'm a bit worried because Stephen and his mates went off to Amsterdam for a weekend and I think he might have . . . you know.

MOLLY   No I don't. Not until you tell me, lovie.

CALLER   I think he might have brought something back.

MOLLY   What, some duty-free booze and cigarettes?

CALLER   No, something more dangerous than that.

MOLLY   Diamonds? Porn mags? Little Dutch cigars?

CALLER   Come on Molly, you must know what I mean.

MOLLY   I'm afraid I don't, lovie. You'll have to be more – how can I put it? – explicit. Don't be afraid to speak your

mind on this programme, we hear all . . .

CALLER I think he may have caught VD.

MOLLY VD?

CALLER That's right. It's put me in a right tizzy.

MOLLY What are the symptoms, lovie?

CALLER Well, I get all nervy and develop a migraine just thinking about it.

MOLLY What are the symptoms of his VD?

CALLER Oh that . . . Well I've noticed this sort of . . . how can I put this . . . sort of . . .

MOLLY Just tell it exactly like it is.

You won't shock us on this programme.

CALLER A sort of green discharge on the end of his willy.

MOLLY Ugh! . . . how revolting!

CALLER Anyway, I'm just wondering what I should do when I am . . . er . . .

MOLLY When you're what, lovie?

CALLER Well, you know, when I'm . . . downstairs . . .

MOLLY In the kitchen?

CALLER No when I'm giving him . . . when I'm . . . er . . .

MOLLY Spit it out, lovie.

CALLER Yes, that's what I thought . . .

SUMMARY
The Do's and Don't's of Safe Sex

DO...

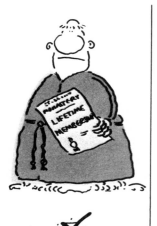

- Wear a condom at all times (even when not having sex)
- Avoid one-night stands
- Avoid hot-dog stands
- Look before you leap
- Leap before you lay
- Stay before you stray

DON'T...

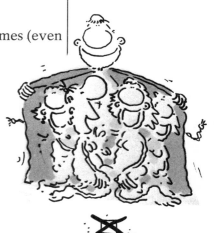

- Bugger around

THE SAFE SEX SURVIVAL GAME

Wait five minutes

START
Are you thinking of having sexual intercourse? — NO / YES

Is your sexual partner demanding money before you do it? — NO / YES

Are you wearing a condom? — NO / YES

Is your partner wearing a condom? — NO / YES

Do you know what a condom is? — NO / YES

Read this book before you begin

Put on a condom, rubber gloves, protective head-gear, boots and apron.

Have you asked your partner if he/she/it, is carrying any sexually transmitted diseases, demanding if necessary medical records and references — NO / YES

Well do so

Find another sexual partner

Have you still got a sexual partner — YES / NO

Have you used this condom before? — NO / YES

Was it good? — NO / YES

Have sexual intercourse

Find another condom

Backword

Well, we hope we have had a little fun with this book, but do remember that the importance of safe sex is serious, deadly serious. Meanwhile there are a few other books you may be interested in reading . . .

More Joys of Safe Sex II by Dr Michael J. Bulstrode and Molly Blackburn.
> *A further penetrating look at the perils of inter-personal relationships.*

Safe Sex, The Early Years by Dr Michael J. Bulstrode, with Molly Blackburn.
> *Safe sex for the under-fives.*

Safe Sex, the Moral Dimension by the Rev. Adabongi Bulstrode and Sister Mary Blackburn.
> *The new puritan morality is explored with full-colour illustrations of sexual practices that might once again be considered improper.*

Confessions of a Club 18–30 Holiday Courier by (Big) Dickie Bulstrode
> *What really goes on when the young get away from it all, and have it away in the sun.*